MW00713816

The Dash Diet CookbooK

Wholesome Recipes for Flavorful Low-Sodium Meals. The Complete Dash Diet Cooking Guide for Beginners to Lower Blood Pressure and Improve Your Health.

KATE DAVIS GREEN

© Copyright 2020 - All rights reserved.

This document is geared towards providing exact and reliable information concerning the topic and issue covered. The publication is sold with the idea that the publisher is not required to render accounting, officially permitted or otherwise qualified services. If advice is necessary, legal or professional, a practiced individual in the profession should be ordered.

From a Declaration of Principles which was accepted and approved equally by a Committee of the American Bar Association and a Committee of Publishers and Associations.

In no way is it legal to reproduce, duplicate, or transmit any part of this document in either electronic means or printed format. Recording of this publication is strictly prohibited, and any storage of this document is not allowed unless with written permission from the publisher. All rights reserved.

The information provided herein is stated to be truthful and consistent, in that any liability, in terms of inattention or otherwise, by any usage or abuse of any policies, processes, or directions contained within is the sole and utter responsibility of the recipient reader. Under no circumstances will any legal liability or blame be held against the publisher for any reparation, damages, or monetary loss due to the information herein, either directly or indirectly.

Respective authors own all copyrights not held by the publisher.

The information herein is offered for informational purposes solely and is universal as so. The presentation of the data is without a contract or any guarantee assurance.

The trademarks that are used are without any consent, and the publication of the trademark is without permission or backing by the trademark owner. All trademarks and brands within this book are for clarifying purposes only and are owned by the owners themselves, not affiliated with this document.

Disclaimer

All intellect contained in this book is given for enlightening and instructive purposes as it were. The creator isn't in any capacity responsible for any outcomes or results that radiate from utilizing this material. Worthwhile endeavors have been made to give data that is both precise and viable. However, the creator isn't oriented for the exactness or use/misuse of this data

TABLE OF CONTENTS

INTRODUCTION

"Health is a state of complete physical, mental and social well-being, and not merely the absence of disease or infirmity."—**Heave**

While the new century unfolds, society faces unprecedented opportunities and challenges. More than ever, the world is united through the Internet, mobile phones and other modern technologies. Around the same time, at an all-time high are the threat of terrorism and nuclear coercion, the proliferation of new infectious diseases and epidemics, and the spread of cancer, heart disease, and other chronic ills. Our children and grandchildren may inherit a hard-to-inhabit globally warmed planet.

Researchers have always been at the forefront of the movement for the last half-century to foster personal and planetary health and peace. Expert, originating from the traditional Greek words for "great life," helps people to take responsibility for their own safety and happiness by harmonization with nature and the universe. Eating a healthy diet of natural foods based on whole grains, peas, beans, sea vegetables and fruits in compliance with the seasons, climate and other environmental factors is the most effective way for doing so.

A healthy diet would help both the world and the people it feeds, according to the environmentalists. Organically growing grains and vegetables as our staple crops instead of animal feeds reduce our reliance on fossil fuels, pesticides and other pollutants, improve the soil's fertility and contribute to cleaner air and water.

Sometimes our minds and our bodies will seem like they are working on two different wavelengths: sometimes your body asks you to take a nap while your brain knows that you still have work to do, or your belly just begs for a candy bar while your brain knows better. Once it comes to our mood, however, our food choices and emotions go hand in hand more often than you would think.

Although a greasy plate of fries or a sugary snack can temporarily relieve a bad mood, a drive-thru rarely does away with long-term happiness. Fortunately, there are plenty of foods with proven mood-enhancing benefits that can help you make every bite happier and safer.

HEALTHY DIET
What is a healthy diet?

Eating a balanced diet is not about rigid limitations, staying unrealistically slim or depriving yourself of the food you enjoy. It's about feeling fantastic, having more time, enhancing your health, and boosting your mood, instead.

It does not have to be overly difficult to eat healthily. For all the contradictory eating and dietary recommendations, you feel confused out there; you are not alone. It seems you will find someone claiming the exact opposite with any expert who tells you a particular food is good with you. The fact is that while it has been shown that certain specific foods or nutrients have a beneficial impact on mood, the most important thing is your overall dietary pattern. The foundation of a balanced diet would be to replace processed food, whenever possible, with real food. Eating food that is as close to nature as possible will make a big difference in the way you think, look, and feel.

HEALTHY NUTRITIONAL HABIT

A habit is that which is learned through repetition. If we talk about nutritional habits, they are those that constitute an eating pattern or what is the same, the usual diet. Healthy habits help prevent food-related illnesses such as type 2 diabetes mellitus, obesity, hypertension, and cardiovascular disease.

A healthy diet, therefore, is one that allows you to maintain the correct functioning of the body continuously and habitually.

Healthy eating habits must include a varied, balanced diet that provides us with the necessary energy and adequate nutrients to stay healthy. But not only the choice of food influences, but also the way of preparing them. We must choose healthy culinary techniques such as cooking or baking and avoid methods such as frying.

Often a lack of time or comfort leads us to make unhealthy food choices when we shop. Within a healthy diet, highly processed foods, confectionery and industrial sweets, salty snacks, soft drinks and an endless number of foods that are increasingly abundant in our pantries must be reduced as much as possible.

One of the things I like to teach the most is the importance of having in our house an excellent healthy pantry that makes it easy for us to prepare multiple easy and tasty recipes.

How to improve your food habits?

To improve your eating habits, you don't need to be hard on yourself. Ensure you follow a proven guide and not make too sudden changes all by yourself. Set small goals that you can achieve. When significant changes in diet are made, the body usually reacts, generating stress and anxiety. If you want your changes to last, adopt good habits, and a healthy lifestyle.

To be successful in improving eating habits, you must be convinced that you want to do it and take the first step. Once you have started, you will see how it becomes easier for you.

These are some of the actions you should take to improve your habits and transform them into a new lifestyle.

Eat Calm and Chew Slowly

Enjoy the moment of the meal, without haste and regrets. Do not eat in front of the television or on the phone. Both proper chewing and the time we spend eating will help us to have better digestions and to feel satiated enough.

Reduce the Consumption of Sugar, Salt and Saturated Fats

Avoid eating highly processed foods that are high in sugar, salt, and fat and replace them with natural, low-processed foods. Reduce the consumption of soft drinks, packaged juices, snacks and industrial sweets.

Increase in Plant Food Consumption

When I recommend increased consumption of plant-based foods, I am not just referring to fruits and vegetables. We must also increase the consumption of legumes, nuts, seeds and whole grains.

Set A Timetable for Eating

Carrying an order in meals will facilitate the process of changing habits. A disordered diet favours cravings, binge eating and poor choices when eating food.

EATING HABITS

"Eating is a necessity, but eating intelligently is an art."

FORMAT OF MEALS

1. Take time for your meals every day.
    - Sit down to eat your meals or snacks without doing other things.
    - Allow adequate time for your meals. Eat slowly and chew well.
    - Stop eating three hours before bedtime. Eat-in an orderly manner.
    - Avoid mixing foods in the same mouthful.
2. Set your daily schedule.
    - Rise early and go to sleep before midnight. Keep your mealtimes regular.
3. Diet: Content and Quality of Meals.
    - Eat two or three complete and nutritionally balanced meals every day.
    - Plan every meal around cooked grains and grain products. Complete and balance every meal with one to two vegetable dishes.

4. Make your daily life activities.

- Walk for thirty minutes every day.
- Give yourself a daily body rub.
- Cultivate and take time for hobbies.
- Life-related exercise provides the most benefit for lasting health.

5. Create a more natural environment.

- Surround yourself with green plants, especially in the bedroom, the kitchen, the bathrooms and office or workspace.
- Wear pure cotton clothing next to your skin.
- Use natural materials such as wood, cotton, silk and wool in your home.

6. Make your practice work.

- Keeping to the format of the meal improves your ability to make healthier food choices.
- Keep a daily record of your meals to help you become more objective about your practice.
- Cultivate the spirit of health.
- Be open, curious and endlessly appreciative of all of life. Learn to be adaptable and flexible in your practice to manifest the excellent result.
- Develop a strong will, habit and the determination to create your own health.
- Create a good quality network support and learn how to cook very well. Be accurate in your practice.

Cooking styles

Try to use a wide variety of cooking styles when you prepare your meals. For daily use, I recommend pressure-cooking, boiling, blanching, steaming, steaming with kombu seaweed, soup-making, stewing, quick sautéing with water or oil, sautéing and simmering, pressing and pickling.

When planning your meals, select foods within the following categories:

whole grains, soups, vegetables, beans, sea vegetables, special foods and beverages. Use different cooking methods from the above list. Keep in mind that it's best not to pressure cook vegetables. Start with those cooking styles that are familiar. If possible, take macrobiotic or natural foods cooking classes. Read cookbooks to inspire and teach you.

Vegetables can be cut in various ways. Try slicing them into rounds or half-moons. You can cut the slices straight across or on the diagonal, and you can vary the thickness of the slices. Different methods have subtly different effects on the flavour and appearance of whatever dish you prepare. Vary the kinds of seasoning and condiments you use. Use different seasonings in dishes you are familiar with and take note of how just a small change in the seasoning of a dish can produce a big difference in taste.

Try seasoning of that same dish with a little more or less of what you usually use. The type and amount of seasoning will each bring out different aspects of flavour and can subtly alter the consistency of a dish. Some seasonings firm up a dish, so to speak, while others have a softening effect. It's important to vary the cooking time of vegetables. Most of us could use more lightly cooked vegetables in our diet.

What do I mean by a lightly cooked vegetable? It's one that makes a crunchy sound when you bite into it. The sound should be audible to someone sitting next to you. No sound means the vegetable is overcooked. Include a combination of well-cooked and lightly cooked vegetable dishes weekly.

Experiment with cooking times. Cook familiar dishes a little longer or for a little less time. And, don't forget that pickles, pressed and raw salad is part of the macrobiotic diet. Try varying the intensity of the flame when you cook. The same dish can taste quite different depending on whether it's been cooked slowly or quickly. Many people use too much fire when cooking. It seems to be a natural tendency to turn the flame up as high as possible whether it's needed or not. Excessive use of a high flame in your cooking may make you nervous or irritable. Use a medium flame when you want to bring something to a boil. If necessary, you can always turn it up at the end of cooking. You will feel calmer and steadier as a result. Vary the combination of dishes you use in meals. Change just one dish, and you have added a new meal to your repertoire. And vary the combination of vegetables, grains, beans and seasonings you use in your dishes. Cook your food a little longer in the winter for warming, energizing effect.

Cooking food a bit less in the summer will produce a cooling and relaxing effect. Try to create a variety of colour, taste and consistency in your meals. Variety means using many different ingredients from each of the different categories, changing the method of preparation and changing the combinations of food. Imagine what the meal will look like on the plate; imagine how it will taste. Remember that variety creates interest and satisfaction. And, never forget that food is meant to be both nourishing and delicious.

First considerations:

- Grains and vegetables together form the basis of complete and balanced nutrition.
- All food has protein. You do not need to make a special effort to increase protein in your diet. It is nearly impossible to become protein deficient.
- A variety of vegetable foods provides the most abundant and well-balanced nutrition available: minerals, including calcium, proteins, carbohydrates, fats, including omega 3, and vitamins, including vitamin C.
- Beans and fish may be included in the same meal.
- Seitan, a wheat gluten product, maybe cooked with grains or beans.
- When planning your daily meals, try to follow the order below:
- Always decide on the grain or grain product first.
- Then choose the vegetable dish or dishes that complement and harmonize the grain.
- Next, decide on the soup to further complete the meal.
- Last, supplement with foods from the other categories, mainly beans, sea vegetables, seeds, nuts, fish, fruit, snacks, desserts, sweets and beverages, if you choose.
- Use these guidelines, whether you are eating at home or out.

Questions to ask when planning every meal:

- What grains or grain products do I want?
- What vegetable dishes do I want?
- Will they be freshly prepared or leftover?

Questions to ask every day:

- What soup shall I have today?
- Do I include brown rice in one of my meals today?
- Am I including a variety of well-cooked, and lightly cooked?

When planning your daily meals, try to follow the order below:

- Always decide on the grain or grain product first.
- Then choose the vegetable dish or dishes that complement and harmonize the grain.
- Next, decide on the soup to further complete the meal.
- Last, supplement with foods from the other categories, mainly beans, sea vegetables, seeds, nuts, fish, fruit, snacks, desserts, sweets and beverages, if you choose.
- Use these guidelines whether you are eating at home or out

HABITS THAT LEAD A HEALTHY LIFE AND INCREASES YOUR PRODUCTIVITY

Healthy diet habit to be more productive.

To be live happy, we want to be productive, and for this, we need to follow a proven healthy diet method.

Do you want to achieve a better result in your day to day activity? This proven diet will help make this possible. Follow the habits that I present below, and I am very confident that your productivity will be multiplied exponentially.

1. Fill the energy tanks with adequate fuel

The quality of carbohydrates is paramount. The complex carbohydrates, found in starchy vegetables and whole grains, are linked to a healthier weight and a reduced risk of type 2 diabetes and heart disease.

The body finds it difficult to break down complex carbohydrates, which is good since they are slowly digested, so the absorption of sugars also occurs gradually.

The increases in blood sugar and insulin levels are moderate enough that we do not store body fat. Also, these carbohydrates are good for the intestinal flora, as they help strengthen the immune system and reduce inflammation.

Finally, most foods that contain complex carbohydrates are also high in fibre, which regulates blood sugar and helps you feel full.

2. Refined carbohydrates

In contrast, refined carbohydrates, such as white bread, juices, cookies, and chips, have the opposite effect. They raise blood sugar, causing insulin levels to skyrocket. They also produce substances that cause intestinal inflammation.

If you opt for refined carbohydrates, metabolic malfunction, high triglycerides, obesity and other accompanying diseases are almost guaranteed.

Obviously, your productivity will decrease. So better opt for complex carbohydrates.

Eating a healthy diet does not mean eliminating carbohydrates but choosing the good ones.

3. Size does matter

"Although someone may find it a little funny," I'm sorry to tell you that size does matter. Imagine that it's time for lunch at work. "You've gone to the fridge and" crossed out" You have taken out the salad bowl your mother has prepared for you. You start eating, and when you have noticed you have eaten almost 3/4 of a kilo of salad that added to the water and the fruit has caused you not to be able to shake.

Yes, you are eating healthy, but friend, you have eaten a lot of food. Your head is going to be more concerned with complaining about how bad you feel about eating "Pecha" than being productive at work.

Obviously, your productivity will be reduced after lunch. So, you know, eat the salad, but make it a normal portion. That you follow a healthy diet does not mean that you have to put yourself up to the very handles.

4. Don't use lunch to finish unfinished business

Perhaps you think that catching up on emails or other chores during lunch will help you get ahead. Instead, what will happen is that you will not rest. You will enter the vicious circle of being continuously tired.

As a result, workers who skip lunch are more stressed and less productive than those who don't skip it.

You know, relax and enjoy doing what you 'can't do while working. Eat healthily, read a book, hang out with a friend or partner, or exercise

5. Hydrate properly

We all know that to improve and maintain enviable health, we have to exercise, follow a healthy diet and rest.

The other element that is usually forgotten is hydration. Well, a gross mistake. Hydration is vital for both physical and mental performance.

Our brains are made up of approximately 70% water while our bodies are made up of around 50-75% water, depending on age and sex. Therefore, it is not surprising that not being well hydrated can affect both our attitude at work and our performance.

Other research has shown that even a reduction in hydration levels of as little as 2% of body weight can negatively influence mood, fatigue, and alertness levels.

In other words, water also has a lot to do with productivity.

Checklist

To ensure a proper daily intake of water:

- Start the day with two glasses of water.
- Drink on your way to work.
- Put a bottle of water in your job bag.

This will ensure you drink throughout the day. Use urine colour as an indicator of hydration. It must be transparent. The darker, your urine the worse hydrated you are.

If you have a headache, feel tired, or have any symptoms related to dehydration, start by drinking a glass of water.

For me, hydration is a fundamental part of a happy and healthy lifestyle. And of course, a productive day.

KEEPING RECORDS OF THE PREVIOUS DIET

Good eating habits, steps one and two, are the controlling factors in good health. The point here is that by keeping to the Format of Meals, we automatically have clear guidelines as to wise food choices under any circumstances, whether we're eating at home, in a restaurant, or on an aero plane. As I said earlier, the biggest mistake most people make is to **focus on Diet:** Content and Quality rather than on Eating Habit**s: Format of Meals**. Eating Habits are what keep us on track

Eating home versus eating out

Food choices that are clear when we eat at home can seem murky when we eat out. When we're at home; we can choose the highest quality organically grown short grain brown rice, organic vegetables, the best quality miso and so on. If we are at the mercy of a mediocre restaurant, we might order white rice and steamed broccoli (possibly even frozen). The quality is lower, yes, but the Format is intact. We have a grain and a vegetable on our plate. Quality can always be adjusted up or down, depending on where we find ourselves. Of course, the degree of adjustment depends on our condition. We must ask: "What can my health afford at this time? How liberal can I be?"

As simple as this might sound, most people see little or no connection between meals at home and meals outside the home. At home, they take care to make good choices, but when they eat out, they often throw away the guidelines, meaning the Format of Meals and choose whatever appeals to them. This is a severe mistake. The Format is what helps us maintain our direction toward health. If, however, we believe Content and Quality are more critical than Format, and we 'can't get organic short-grain rice, the temptation is to abandon the Format as well. Once we create separation in our minds between what we eat at home and what we eat outside, it follows that we begin to see food in terms of black and white. We think, "I ate something I shouldn't have," I'm off the diet, I'm in trouble, I can never eat out, this is too hard. But, if we focus on the Format wherever we are, we will automatically make the wisest choices possible, and we will continue to move in the direction of health.

The second biggest mistake Let's look at maintaining the direction toward health from another angle; structure (another word for Format) versus variety. The second biggest mistake most people make is to allow the structure, which should be tight, to become loose. Once that happens, the need for variety diminishes and eventually changes to a pattern of repetition, a pattern that directs us away from health. If the legs of a table are loose, the table can be said to have a shaky structure. It can barely support itself. If we remove the legs altogether, the table will collapse completely. Or to use Nature's model once again, the sun rises and sets every day, a phenomenon that is part of the structure of the universe. If the sun" doesn't rise or set, it's all over for the planet. In the same way, once we let the structure or Format go, we set ourselves on a path away from health.

Here are the main danger signals:

- You don't sit down and take time for your meals.
- You do other things while eating.
- Your mealtimes become irregular.
- You stop having a grain and vegetable with every meal. How does this work?

Let's say you want to have lunch at twelve-thirty, no later than one o'clock, but you're too busy to eat. By the time you do eat, your appetite is completely altered because your blood sugar has fallen. Low blood sugar means that to feel satisfied, either you have to eat more than usual—in other words, overeat—or you have to have something sweet. It follows that once having eaten a late lunch; you have no appetite for dinner at the regular time. If you keep to your regular dinnertime but eat less than usual, an hour or two later" you'll want a snack. Or, instead of dinner at six, let's say you decide to eat at eight-thirty. Either way, you won't have three full hours between dinner and bedtime since you have to go to bed at a reasonable hour in order to get up early the next morning. You "don't sleep very well that night (no one sleeps well on a full stomach). It's challenging to get up the next morning and, when you do drag yourself out of bed, you" don't feel refreshed. You can see how one change in the structure or Format inevitably leads to another and how, in the end, these changes will lead you away from health. Although having a grain and vegetable with every meal comes under the heading of Diet, there is an overlap with Format. The meal you sit down to eat must qualify as a meal, meaning it must contain a grain or grain product and a vegetable. When you stop having both a grain and a vegetable with every meal, most commonly that meal is breakfast, and it's the vegetable that disappears from the plate. If "you've reached this stage, you can pretty much assume" you've begun to lose your direction. You're getting way off track.

Balance and imbalance perpetuate themselves

One of the guiding principles of life is that balance perpetuates itself. And, as you might suspect, imbalance perpetuates itself as well. As you let go of more and more of the structure, you start to feel more and more pressure. You might believe the build-up of stress comes from having to visit the market, prepare and cook the food or from the pressure of having to eat at a regular time— but I don't think so. I think the reverse is true. The usual pattern is that you feel rushed, so you begin to rush your meals. The more we rush our meals, the more rushed we feel. Sitting down and taking time for meals, actually eases pressure. If you think of a meal as a time for recharging, reorienting and regaining balance, if no matter how stressed you feel you take the time to sit down, eat slowly and chew well when you finish eating you will feel refreshed and calm. Any decisions you make in this frame of mind are bound to be wiser than those made under pressure.

Some people find it helpful to think of chewing as a form of meditation, somewhat like breathing practices. The result in both cases is heightened mental and emotional clarity and a feeling of deep calm. Remember, it's essential to come to the table prepared to chew. Before you sit down, ask yourself. "What are my priorities?" If good health is one of them, then take time for your meal, eat your food slowly and chew it well.

Structure Versus Variety

Let's go back to structure versus variety. I said earlier that when the structure becomes loose, the need for variety diminishes—or we could say, tightens—and eventually, repetition replaces variety altogether. In effect, polarity is reversed. **What do I mean by this?** Let me start with a basic premise: the more we seek variety, the more nutrition we get from our food. If we eat the same few foods over and over again, eventually not much happens. If someone repeats the same thing over and over again,

---

27

yet you stop hearing what is being said. It goes in one ear and out from the other. It's no different with food. In one end and out the other—without much benefit. Unfortunately, often we don't notice that this is happening. 'It's difficult to be aware of what we're eating day-to-day. Food is the closest thing to us, so we don't have the advantage of perspective.

We think we have variety, and we eat blanched, steamed and sauteed vegetables daily; we eat different grains, oatmeal, brown rice, millet, barley where's the repetition in all this? Every morning we have oatmeal and steamed kale; for lunch, we have rice and blanched broccoli and cabbage; for dinner, miso soup, rice with sesame seeds, sautéed mixed vegetables, pressed salad with Nappa cabbage. Isn't that variety? No. It's repetition. Taking several dishes and repeating them day after day after day is repetition. Having blanched broccoli and cabbage every day for lunch is repetition. Having oatmeal for breakfast every morning is repetition. Appetite is stimulated by variety. Variety also creates satisfaction. If we lack variety in both ingredients and preparation, we don't feel satisfied with our food, and so we overeat at mealtimes and snack before bed.

Highlights:

- Good eating habits, steps one and two, are the controlling factors in good health.
- Good eating habits increase your ability to make healthy choices.
- When travelling or eating out, keep to the format of grains and vegetables as the basis of a meal. Quality can be adjusted up or down.
- White rice or commercial pasta is a better choice than going without a grain.
- Commercial vegetable soup is a better choice than no soup at all.

KEEP TRACK OF YOUR DAILY DIET OBJECTIVE

Underlying everything in this book so far is the fundamental question, how do we keep moving in the direction of health? Keeping a menu book or a journal, if you prefer to call it that—is the best way I know of. It's challenging to be aware of what we're doing day to day, especially about diet. As I've said before, food is the closest thing to us, so it's hard to be objective. The power of a menu book is that it lets you see if you are really getting enough variety. Enter the date, time and menu for every meal, snack or nibble that passes your lips along with a brief comment on how you felt that day. Review your menu book every so often and reflect on its contents. It's difficult to be objective when you are entering information. Objectivity comes later.

In this way, you will know whether or not you are getting variety. Keeping a daily menu book takes the guesswork out of tracking the changes in your health. (It's not necessary to include recipes, although you may if you wish.) Your menu book can be as simple or as detailed as you care to make it. Some people keep track of their daily functions as well as their daily food—bowel movements, bedtime, sleep patterns, moods, and so on. Looking back, you can see how you were feeling physically, mentally and emotionally on any given day. Then you can begin to correlate what you ate or did on a particular day with how you felt that day.

For instance: I did this, and I felt really good—my thinking was clear, I ate this and I didn't feel very well, I did this, and I was irritable, I did that, and I was exhausted. You can't learn this sort of thing in school. How certain foods, patterns and behaviours affect, you can only be self-taught. If you write just a sentence or two every day, that should be enough to jog your memory and help you discover whether you are really doing what you think you're doing. I 'can't stress enough the importance of keeping a menu book. It's one way to measure how serious your commitment is to improving and strengthening your health. I must confess I've never really kept a menu book but, in the past, during the years when I was teaching several times a week, I kept a kind of journal. I entered the outline of every class I gave along with some comments, no matter how often I teach the same topic. It's interesting to look back over these journals. There are times when I thought my condition was good, and my thinking orderly, but my record shows otherwise. Or, looking back at other periods when my notes indicate that my condition was off, I can see by the outline of my class that my thinking was obvious and orderly. The point is that when you're in the throes of doing something, it's nearly impossible to be objective. But when you look back, you can often see the truth. One final comment on this point: You might think you don't need to do this, you're an experienced cook, you" don't need to improve your cooking.

Let me assure you that even experienced, and longtime food cooks keep menu books. I can guarantee that if you keep one, your practice will improve, so as your cooking. Objectivity is the key. You can see where you been lagging or gone overboard.

Highlights:

- Keep a hard or spiral-bound book in your kitchen to record your menus and snacks.
- Keep notes on your activities, symptoms and general feelings.
- Refer back to previous days, weeks and months to see any patterns that emerge from your practice.
- Keeping a daily menu book is one of the best ways to improve your practice and discover your mistakes.
- Such a journal allows you to evaluate your practice and its benefits more objectively

Habits and healthy food?

A change in habits that leads to a healthy lifestyle is going to provide us with numerous benefits. Within a healthy lifestyle, food is one of the three fundamental pillars. The other two are physical exercise and sleep.

BENEFIT OF HEALTHY DIET GUIDELINE

Healthy diet is a vital key to living a happy and productive life. Below are proven benefit that follows keeping track of your diet.

Have More Energy: An adequate supply of calories and nutrients provides us with enough energy to maintain the activities we carry out. If we eat empty calories or with a poor supply of nutrients, we will feel tired and lack energy.

Protect Cardiovascular Health: An adequate consumption of fats will help improve the lipid profile, reduce cholesterol and improve cardiovascular health.

Improve Your Quality Of Life: Adequate weight and the absence of food-related illnesses greatly improves the quality of life.

Get Greater Well-Being: A proper and orderly eating pattern helps you feel good not only physically, but also emotionally.

Prevent Diseases: Food-related diseases, such as obesity, diabetes 2 and hypertension, can be prevented and can also be improved and even reversed with a change inhabits.

Improve Your Physical Aspect: It is well known that a balanced and varied diet helps maintain a good weight and also improves the appearance of both skin and hair.

MENTAL CLARITY

"ill-health, of the body or of mind, is defeat. Health alone is a victory. Let all men, if they can manage it, contrive to be healthy."
—Thomas Carlyle

Mental state and food

The influence of food on our mental well-being is based on different complex element interplay. Not only certain foods can have a positive effect on our happiness but our mental state play a major role on our happiness.

Factors such as the quality of the food and the enjoyment experience while eating, as well as how it is consumed, is also important.

Serotonin is a happiness enhancer

The messenger substance serotonin is one of the decisive factors in increasing happiness. In addition to our mood, this also controls the body temperature, the sleep rhythm and the sex drive. In higher concentrations, serotonin, also known as" the happiness hormone", can have a positive effect on a person's mood. On the other hand, if the concentration of serotonin in the body is too low, this will cloud our mood.

The messenger substance can be absorbed through food. However, what is more, important is the body's own serotonin production in the brain, which can be promoted through a balanced diet.

Increase in serotonin concentration

Nevertheless, a balanced diet can indirectly promote the body's production of serotonin. The concentration of serotonin is increased by increasing the intake of substances which produce serotonin.

The organism needs the following "ingredients" to synthesize the messenger substance:

The basic building block tryptophan, the precursor of serotonin, is an amino acid that is found in foods such as fish, milk and soy products, but also in Brazil nuts, plums, pineapple or spelled. Incidentally, the intake of tryptophan is slowed down by eating protein-rich food, so it is advisable to take a low-protein diet.

Carbohydrates are crucial because they promote the transport of tryptophan and its absorption into the brain. Pasta, potatoes, or sugary foods like chocolate are rich in carbohydrates.

Magnesium can be found in broccoli, cocoa or soy products, for example. For a stable feeling, you need a highly varied, balanced diet.

Soul Food: These foods make you happy

Foods that contain several of the ingredients required for the production of serotonin are particularly popular as soul food. These include, for example:

- Dried fruits such as dates and figs
- dark chocolate
- whole-grain products
- Bananas
- Avocados
- nuts

MENTAL EATING
Emotional Healing Through food

Food is an excellent tool to be able to do a detox on a physical, mental, emotional and spiritual level that will lead us to some benefits that are closely related to emotional healing. Cleaning and eliminating toxins from our body and continuing with healthy lifestyle habits help us to have more mental clarity. This helps us to be more aware of our emotions, to detect better what happens to us physically and emotionally, to meet again with our deepest desires and needs and to reset our organs. Thanks to all this, it will be inevitable that later emotional changes will come, progressively, deeper.

Research shows many people who have done an online or face-to-face program with an expert on how something magical has happened as a result of changing eating habits and lifestyle. They have made the decision and the necessary actions to change everything that no longer works in their life.

Thanks to the first changes in diet, other very profound and, above all, essential ones have followed because they were the root of their bad eating habits and harmful behaviours with food. In fact, this is what happened to me.

Eating highly nutritious and healthy meal helps us to become aware of what is working in our lives and what is not. But this does not mean that we solve what we must solve. From this realization, the path of emotional healing begins, which most of the time, we cannot do on our own or only with just any food. Still, we must resort to a professional who guides us, accompanies us and tools to learn to live the life from another point of view. I will never be tired of repeating that there are **two ways of living: one is from fear,** which leads us to suffer anxiety, cravings, emotional hunger, panic attacks, obsession with food, toxic relationships with others and with ourselves, negative thoughts, constant guilt, and stress, while the **other is from LOVE**, that is, where we have healthy relationships that add us, positive thoughts, we observe ourselves with curiosity, we are kind to ourselves and others, we put aside criticism to be tolerant and flexible, and anxiety, guilt, stress and exhaustion dissipate from our life.

When we eat healthy food, we begin to experience more energy and are more proactive and co-creators of our reality. Our paradigm of what life is and how we relate to it changes. We stop seeing ourselves as victims of what happens to us to become, and we take responsibility for it. We appreciate everything that happens because it does it so that we learn something, but also because we know that from the moment it happens to us, it means that Life is already has accepted it. We find our purpose, and we know our value contribution and, ultimately, we know ourselves. This self-knowledge is what we need to stop acting in a self-destructive way, to listen to what our body really needs and to heal ourselves emotionally. If we don't know each other, we can't accept ourselves. If we don't accept ourselves, we don't love each other. If we don't love each other, we don't respect each other. If we don't respect ourselves, we don't eat what really nourishes us from the inside out. It is that easy and yet so complicated at first because we are very entangled in our mind and our emotions, and we live disconnected from our essence.

Emotional healing and healthy eating

For me, emotional healing and healthy food go hand in hand as the combination of the two leads to happiness. A person who eats healthy, energetic and nutritious food will become happy. Heal their emotions more quickly and easily because they are more awake, more present, more aware of everything and will not be able or will not want to close their eyes to their reality.

And an emotionally healthy person will easily eat foods that truly nourish them and will not resort to false foods that take away their energy. Put them in a bad mood, cause physical ill health, or need to cover or evade with food. That is, you will not put your well-being in danger by false food. Because if we love, accept and respect everything else that flows: we eat beneficial foods, we want to move our bodies, we interact with people who are in the same energy, we get the job that fits our way of being, We appreciate each day. And we are at peace with life and our environment.

To achieve good emotional health, we must pay attention to our physical body. We need to nourish our body with real foods that do not cause an alteration in our intestines since millions of bacteria are found in them with a direct relationship to our emotional health. Research has unveiled that human studies have already been carried out in which the microbiota (intestinal flora) of healthy people is compared with that of others who have a particular disease. It has been seen that modifying the intestinal ecosystem or its functions can reduce anxiety states. People with gastrointestinal disorders, such as irritable bowel syndrome, has been observed that they have problems such as depression or even anxiety. In these patients with mental disorders, half have been observed to have issues with the digestive system.

Our emotional bodywork require adequate attention. This can be achieved by correcting what is preventing us from shining. For our mental body to change those beliefs and thoughts that are limiting us and to our spiritual body to find our contribution of value and our purpose, I invite you now to reflect on what it is that you really seek to heal by looking within. What is stopping you from living out of love?

In the meantime, also write in a notebook what is the small change in habits or diet that you will do to start this healing journey that started HERE today. You have just made a commitment to yourself knowing that emotional healing is the result of a process of self-knowledge that is not done overnight and that no one will do for you. So **CONGRATULATIONS!**

Foods, in addition to it being tasty, give us energy, are the fuel for our body and comfort us in stressful situations. But can food improve your memory or help you be smarter? Several kinds of research have shown that certain foods have nutrients that can strengthen our memory or concentration capacity.

In the 1990s, researchers found that when adults listen to music by Wolfgang Amadeus Mozart, they perform better on intelligence tests. Numerous studies have been done since then on foods to know which ones increase intelligence.

Certain foods can help boost your brain power, clear your mental confusion, and make your thinking skills quick.

To do what I have done to feel at peace and tranquillity with what you eat, here is a list of those foods that will help you increase your mental clarity, overcome anxiety, stress, insomnia, recover menses or heal intestinal dysbiosis and the ability to think so that you include them in your daily diet:

1. Bluefish (Salmon, Sardines, Horse Mackerel)

More than half of the brain mass is made up of lipids, and more than 65% of these are fatty acids that belong to the Omega family. These fats are vital for the production and development of brain cells, maintaining the fluidity of the cell membrane. They also play an important role in the activity of neurons. Fatty fish like salmon, tuna, and fresh sardines contain Omega 3 fats that help brain cells interrelate with each other. Make it an habit to eat at least two servings of fish a week. Fish contains phosphorus and iodine, both of which are important for brain work.

2. Dairy Products (Milk, Cheese, Cream)

Dairy products are especially useful for our brain. Lack of fat can be the reason for various unpleasant diseases, for example, multiple sclerosis. What's more, protein, calcium, vitamin D and magnesium found in dairy products, play an important role in stimulating brain activity.

3. Lean Red Meat

A study published in 2011 found that women with healthy iron levels performed better on mental tasks and finished faster than those with low iron levels. This metal helps transport oxygen throughout the body and to the brain. Lack of iron in the diet can reduce the blood's ability to transport oxygen, decreasing the amount delivered to the brain. Not taking enough iron can also cause problems such as lack of energy, poor concentration, and tiredness. Low-fat meat is an excellent source of iron and zinc, minerals important for the brain's cognitive function.

4. The Blanquillos

A good source of iron is egg yolk. Eggs contain phospholipids and lecithin, necessary to build the membrane of brain cells. In terms of increasing intelligence, its value lies mainly in its proteins. Eggs are in fact rich in amino acids, vital in the production of the main neurotransmitters.

5. Leafy Vegetables (Spinach, Lettuce, Broccoli)

Studies show that people who take more vitamin C do better on tests of attention and memory. Experts suggest eating at least 5 servings of vegetables and fruit a day, but eating a variety is the key. All leafy greens are rich in vitamin B9 or folate, which is believed to play an active role in the development of nervous tissue of the fetus and also in the renewal of blood cells. Choose spinach, lettuce, watercress, broccoli, or different types of herbs Rosemary has certain flavonoids, especially in its aroma, that stimulate memory and concentration by increasing cerebral blood flow.

6. Legumes (Lentils, Soybeans, Beans, Beans, Chickpeas)

Legumes are very impotant in our diet. To fuel your brain and at the same time keeping your blood sugar levels stable, make it an habit to eat at least two servings of legumes a day. The brain is said to be glucose-dependent. This means that the brain only uses glucose for fuel. Our brain consumes more than five grams per hour but does not know how to store it. That is why the brain has to be supplied regularly by glucose through the circulatory system. Complex sugars are crucial. Legumes are full of these complex sugars, and their glycemic index is one of the lowest. It really allows the regulation of glucose in the blood and supplies it to the brain without creating a hyperglycemic reaction.

7. Red Berries

Bilberry is rich in antioxidants. Nerve cells are at high risk of oxidative damage and need special antioxidant protection at any time in life. Its ability to send impulses through the body depends on balanced oxygen metabolism, and this balance cannot be achieved without taking antioxidant nutrients. All edible berries are sources of vitamin C, Blackcurrants have three times more vitamin C concentration than kiwi and two times more than citrus. In addition to strengthening the blood ducts and improving circulation, they allow better oxygenation of the brain, and they fight against free radicals that can affect nerve cells, especially brain cells.

8. Avocado

Avocado is almost as good as the blueberry in protecting brain health. Avocado is a fatty fruit, but it is a monounsaturated fat that contributes to healthy blood flow. And healthy blood flow leads to a healthy brain. Avocados also lower blood pressure. It is rich in vitamin E, which is a powerful antioxidant and protects the fatty tissues of the brain from ageing. The absorption of beta carotene and lycopene increases when fresh avocado or avocado oil is added to any salad. However, avocados are high in calories, so it is suggested to eat only 1/2 or 1/4 of an avocado at a daily meal as a garnish.

9. Coffee and Tea

The presence of caffeine molecules gives tea and coffee their true value as a tonic and stimulant. These hot drinks can improve cognitive function and prevent " Alzheimer's disease. A 2011 study found that when researchers gave caffeinated coffee to mice genetically engineered to develop this disease, progression was slower or did not develop. The tea also showed protective effects on the brain. In addition to the high content of antioxidants that help fight free radicals and increase brain activity, tea drinkers perform better on memory tests and information processing.

10. Nuts and Seeds

Walnuts and seeds are a source of vitamin E. Several studies suggest that an adequate intake of vitamin E can help prevent cognitive decline, especially in young age. Adding an ounce, a day of hazelnuts, walnuts, Brazil nuts, almonds, peanuts, sesame seeds, sunflower seeds and flax seeds, among others, is all you need to obtain the recommended daily amount of zinc, essential for the improvement of thinking and memory skills. Regular consumption of niacin-rich foods like peanuts protects against age-related cognitive decline and Alzheimer's disease. Peanut is a source of vitamin E which is an antioxidant that protects the nerve membranes in the brain, prevents the formation of blood clots

By taking care of your diet, you help your body to have a better quality of life.

Eat consciously or mindfully

When you eat lunch, put the phone and possible distractions aside. Concentrate on what you're doing.

Do not check your email, WhatsApp or other social media profile. Take a deep breath, eat slowly and savour the delicious and healthy food that you are having the pleasure of eating.

Enjoy the food, don't gobble up.

Not only the quantity and composition of the food make you feel satisfied. So do sensory aspects like taste, aroma, texture, and colour. If you gobble up the food, you probably 'haven't even noticed that you've eaten. Very soon, you will need to eat again.

Be kind and generous to yourself and forget about everything during meals. If you're going to be stressed or checking things on the phone, your productivity will continue to decrease after lunch. Concentrate and enjoy the food, and there will be time to solve what comes after the break.

If you are the workaholic type, forget about the work completed you will feel more rested and fresher. The productivity battery will be recharged. You've spent it from morning to noon, and you have to reload it for the second part of the day.

Don't ignore hunger

We want to eat healthily and be productive. I don't want you to be confused and believe that to be productive; you have to be slim at all costs even if it leads to starvation.

It is not what I try to convey to you in this book. What I DO want to share with you is that if you eat healthily, you will be happier, and better both physically and mentally. You will rest better; you will have more energy, you will be more positive, you will get sick less. In short, your productivity will be exponentially multiplied.

Eat healthily but don't ignore hunger.

My experience

It has happened to me. There have been times when I have been from 9:00 to 18:00 without trying a bite. I have been seeing patients in consultation and have not even had time to remember to eat.

What do you think happened when 18:00 arrived? Well, I have relaxed. Suddenly the stomach begins to roar, and I devour without control neither on the quantities nor on the quality of the food.

I also have a major headache. And of course, that since 14:00 I have been a living dead, that is, I maintain myself because I have no other choice and I have someone in front of me; otherwise things would change. My performance has dropped in the second half of the day.

Also, when I got home, I ate all that I had not eaten during the day. At about 7:30 p.m. I feel bloated, have indigestion, and the feeling of nausea begins to emerge. I have no desire to do anything and less to continue eating.

This is why I tell you to drink something when your stomach asks you to. Do not ignore it. I don't want you to force yourself to eat but listen to your body. So always have a healthy snack on hand. Some days are chaotic, and these snacks can save your life.

If you have eaten well throughout the day, you will have a much better chance of eating well when you get home. And eating right when you get home means " "you're probably going to wake up happy to do something productive later in the day.

Do not take sugars

Most of people think that fats are to blame for all of "today's food-related disease.

This is not like this. The bad guy in the movie is sugar." Don't demonize fats.

Here I leave you more information about fats that will leave you speechless.

If you include sugars in your diet, you will probably have to fight all day against hunger. Therefore, you will eat more and worse. Your weight and your health problems will increase. Eventually, it will result in a loss of productivity.

Also, I want you to know that the continuous consumption of sugar can lead to:

- Weight gain.
- Insulin resistance.
- Diabetes.
- Obesity.
- Fatty liver.
- Pancreatic cancer.
- Chronic renal failure.
- Arterial hypertension.

- Cardiovascular diseases.
- Addiction.
- Malnutrition
- The appearance of caries.

Possible drop-in sugar

Also, just after taking products rich in sugar, you may experience high energy because of the spike in blood sugar that has occurred.

The problem is that by increasing blood sugar levels, the pancreas secretes insulin to eliminate it. Sugar is pushed by insulin to the liver and muscles, which are probably already loaded with glycogen. This is going to cause this sugar to transform and store as fat.

This will cause a decrease in blood sugar that will give us a crash. I know you would not want this to happen to you. Guess what the body is going to ask you when this happens? Indeed, more sugar.

And what are you doing? Add more sugar, and it would lack more.

It ends up happening what we feared. You have entered a vicious circle from which you cannot escape.

If this happens one day, it has no significant consequences. You probably have not been very productive because you have been more aware of the fight against the sugar-hunger pairing. But there is also no need to give more thought to the head.

On the other hand, if this happens often, you have many ballots that your weight is high. So will the percentage of body fat. And you know what happens when you do not have a healthy diet and we have a flawed body or better said, up to the handle. Yes, your productivity and performance are diminished.

LATE NIGHT HABIT

Last food intake two hours before going to bed. This topic has caused a lot of controversy in recent times.

It has always been thought that at night is when you should least eat. We believe that metabolism slows down, we burn a few calories, and fat accumulation is greater. Instead, other experts think that eating at night helps you lose weight and even sleep better.

The problem is that there is evidence for both situations.

Some studies conclude that the nocturnal metabolic rate is equal to the daytime. On the other hand, other reviews link eating at night with weight gain.

How I go about it?

If you have no choice but to eat at night and late, go ahead. Eat healthy, softly and without overloading yourself. Now, if you have the possibility, avoid it and eat something earlier.

Keep this in mind:

- Melatonin, a hormone that helps us regulate sleep, rises at night to indicate that it is time to sleep. It also reduces the function of different organs, such as those responsible for controlling glucose levels.
- Digestion will cause our body temperature to rise, delaying the onset of sleep. Keep in mind that the decrease in body temperature is another sign that helps us rest.
- If you have gastroesophageal reflux, it is a good idea to eat at least 2 hours before going to bed.

For this reason, you should not leave dinner until the last minute. They are small details that will improve the quality of your rest.

You know, if you rest better you will be much more productive.

If you make a hearty meal at the last minute, you will not rest well; you will have to get up to drink water several times during the night and probably the next day you will wake up with indigestion. You will start the day on the left foot, more worried about your stomach than what awaits you at work.

You will probably choose not to eat breakfast, and you will re-enter the vicious circle of mood swing, poor diet and lost productivity.

CONCLUSIONS

I hope that after reading through this book, everything that I wanted to convey to you has become clear to you. If you follow a healthy diet, you are much more likely to be productive and be happy.

Not only will you be physically better. You will also find yourself psychologically unstoppable. Being physically and psychologically well will exponentially multiply your productivity.

I don't want to say that if you don't eat well, you won't be happy or productive. I mean that **if you take care of what you eat, you are much more likely to happy and more productive.**

I hope this book provides you with enough guidance on how to eat healthily and be more productive.

As productivity is like sport, you can train, improve and optimize in many ways. Here is a list of recipes that make you happy as you prepare and set out to serve them.

HAPPY DIET RECIPES

Almond Meal Pita Chips

Serves: 2–4

Cooking time: 15 minutes

Ingredient:

- 1 1/2 cups of almond meal, plus extra for dusting on rolling pin to prevent sticking
- 1/2 teaspoon of garlic powder
- 1/2 teaspoon of salt
- 1 egg

Instruction

1. Preheat oven to 350°
2. Whisk together almond meal, garlic powder, and salt.
3. Add egg and mix well into a thick batter.
4. Roll or press batter out evenly onto parchment paper to approximately 1/4-inch thickness.
5. Bake for 15 minutes until crisp and golden brown.
6. Break apart into chips.

Sausage Stuffed Mushrooms

Serves: 8 – 10

Cooking time: 50 minutes

Ingredient:

- 2 tablespoons olive oil
- 1 small onion, finely chopped
- 1 garlic clove, minced
- 1 pound of large button or baby Bella mushrooms stems cored out and finely
- chopped for the stuffing mixture
- 1 pound of your favourite sausage casing discarded
- 1 tablespoon red wine vinegar
- 2/3 cup almond meal, plus more for sprinkling
- 1/4 cup of Boursin cheese (the original goat cheese, not the spread)

Instruction:

1. Preheat oven to 325°
2. In a large sauté pan with olive oil heated to medium-high heat.
3. Cook onion until soft, about 3–4 minutes.
4. Add garlic, cook another 1 minute.
5. Add chopped mushroom stems.
6. Cook 4–5 minutes until very soft.
7. Add sausage, browning thoroughly and using a spatula to chop up into small bits.
8. Drain and discard excess fat if necessary.
9. Sprinkle red wine vinegar over sausage.
10. Mix in almond meal evenly.
11. Remove from heat and fold in Boursin cheese until evenly mixed and creamy.
12. Place mushroom caps hollow side up in an 8 x 8 baking pan.

13. Spoon sausage mixture into mushroom caps. Sprinkle additional almond meal on top.
14. Bake at 325°F for 45 minutes, or until mushrooms are cooked, and topping is golden brown. Cool for 10 minutes, then serve.

Kalamata Olive Tapenade

Servers: 2 – 3 cups

Cooking time: 45 seconds

Ingredient:

- 1/3 cup raw pine nuts
- 2 cups pitted kalamata olives
- 2 tablespoons capers, rinsed off
- 2 teaspoons Dijon mustard
- 1/2 teaspoon minced garlic
- 2 tablespoons olive oil
- 1 teaspoon fresh lemon juice
- 2 anchovy fillets, rinsed and dried (optional)

Instruction:

1. In a food processor, blend the pine nuts until they turn into nut butter, about 30–45 seconds.
2. Add the remaining ingredients and pulse until finely chopped, with a chunky paste consistency, about 10 pulses, scraping down the side of the food processor to make sure all ingredients blend nicely.
3. Put in an airtight container and refrigerate overnight to let the flavours take time to settle in. Bring to room temperature before serving.

Prosciutto Wrapped Peaches

Output: 16 – 18 pieces

Ingredient:

- 3 peaches, peeled, pitted, and cut into 1-inch wedges
- 5 slices of prosciutto, sliced lengthwise and into thirds.

instruction

1. Heat a sauté pan to medium-high heat.
2. Place prosciutto-wrapped peaches in a clock formation in your pan, starting with the noon position.
3. This way, you remember where you started when 'it's time to flip each piece.
4. Cook until prosciutto is hardening but is not too crisp.
5. Flip and repeat on each side of the peach wedge.
6. The peach will be warm and slightly gooey on the outside.
7. Serve immediately. Watch your guests "ooh" and "ahh"as the peaches melt in their mouths.

Wrap prosciutto around peach slices, using a toothpick to keep in place if necessary.

Cheese Crisps

Serves: 1

Cooking time: 3 minutes

Ingredient:

- 1/4 cup shredded cheese (cheddar, mozzarella, or Colby Jack)

Instruction:

1. Heat a small sauté pan to medium-high heat
2. spread shredded cheese into a 4-6 circle and fry in a pan, being careful not to burn, until cheese is golden and bubbly.
3. Remove from pan and let cool on a paper towel. Or eat immediately, but please don't burn your mouth.
4. Alternately, place 1/4 cup shredded cheese on a plate.
5. Spread thinly into a 4–6 circle.
6. Microwave 75–90 seconds until the cheese comes out in a cooked, flat disk.
7. Peel the cheese crisp off the plate and let cool until crispy

Tzatziki Dip

Serve: 2 – 3

Cooking time: 10 minutes

Ingredient:

- 5 Persian cucumbers or
- 1 large English cucumber, roughly peeled and chopped
- 1 tablespoon fresh dill 1 garlic clove
- chopped 2 tablespoons lemon juice (about 1/2 a lemon)
- 2 teaspoons salt 2 cups Greek yoghurt
- Salt and pepper for finishing

Instruction:

- Lay cucumber pieces on a flat surface.
- Sprinkle with salt and let sit for 10 minutes to draw out excess water.
- Dab dry with a paper towel. Combine dill, garlic, cucumber, lemon juice, and salt in a food processor or Vitamix.
- Pulse until blended but chunky.
- Pour into a mixing bowl. Whisk in Greek yoghurt, combining well.
- Serve alongside grilled meat and veggies, or as a dip with almond meal pita chips.

Cauliflower Pizza Crust

Serve: (Yields 1 - 10 thin crust)

Cooking time: 20 minutes

Ingredient:

- 2 12-ounce bags of cauliflower florets, stems removed
- 1/4 cup grated parmesan 1/4 cup shredded mozzarella
- 1/2 teaspoon garlic powder 1/2 teaspoon dried oregano
- 1/2 teaspoon dried basil
- 1/2 teaspoon salt
- 1 egg

For the topping: Homemade Pizza Sauce or store-bought without sugar Your choice of meat, veg, cheese, etc.

1. Pulse cauliflower in a food processor until it resembles the texture of couscous. It will have a snowy appearance.
2. In a microwave-safe bowl, cook on high for 3–4 minutes. Let cool. Using cheesecloth, squeeze all excess water out of the cauliflower, then do one final squeeze wrapping a towel around the cheesecloth to make sure all excess water has been removed.
3. Preheat oven to 425°.
4. In a large mixing bowl, mix cauliflower, parmesan, mozzarella, garlic powder, oregano, basil, salt, and egg very evenly and form a dough ball.
5. Cover a baking sheet with parchment paper. Spray it with a light coating of olive oil or coconut oil. Place dough ball in the centre, and press into a circle, about 10–11 inches in diameter and 1/2 inch thick.
6. Bake in the oven for 11–14 minutes until golden brown spots start to cover the surface of the crust. Remove from oven, add your sauce and toppings, and place back in the oven for 5–7 minutes or until cheese topping is melted and bubbly.

SOUPS:

Different dishes of soups can also leave a healthy feeling after eating

Serves: Chicken Sage Soup (4–6)

Cooking time: 20 minutes

Ingredient:

- 1 tablespoon olive oil
- 1 yellow onion, chopped
- 3 stalks celery, chopped
- 2 carrots, peeled and chopped
- 1/2 teaspoon dried oregano
- 1/2 teaspoon dried basil
- 1/2 teaspoon dried thyme
- 1/2 teaspoon onion powder
- 1/2 teaspoon garlic powder
- 12 sage leaves, chopped
- 4 cups chicken broth (or one box if using store-bought)
- 1 rotisserie chicken, light and dark meat pulled or cut into 1/2-inch pieces
- Freshly grated parmesan cheese for garnish

Instruction:

1. In a large Dutch oven pot or Le Creuset, heat olive oil to medium-high heat until shimmering. Sauté onions, celery, and carrots until very soft, about 8–10 minutes.
2. Add in oregano, basil, thyme, onion powder, and garlic powder, mix in well with vegetables.

---

3. Add in sage leaves, cook for an additional 3–5 minutes. Pour in chicken broth. Let come to boil, then reduce to simmer.
4. Add in chicken and cook for 15–20 minutes. Serve immediately and garnish with fresh parmesan cheese.

Homemade Chicken Stock

Serves: 8–10 cups

Cooking time: 4 hours

Ingredient

- 1 roasted chicken carcass
- 8 baby carrots
- 2 celery stalks, chopped twice
- 1 medium onion quartered (you can leave the skin on if you would like to experiment!)
- 1 bay leaf 1 bouquet garni of herbs on hand; I use oregano, thyme, and sage
- 2 teaspoons salt 1 teaspoon fresh pepper
- 1 tablespoon apple cider vinegar
- Enough water to cover the entire chicken in a large stockpot

Instruction:

1. Place all ingredients in a stockpot.
2. Bring to a boil, then turn down and let simmer 3–4 hours.
3. Drain through a colander, and let cool for a 1/2 hour.
4. Pour stock through a strainer to remove remaining debris.
5. Pour into freezer ware and freeze.

Albondigas Kale Soup

Serves: 6–8

Cooking time: 20 minutes

Meatballs

Ingredient

- 1 pound 80/20 ground beef (I use ground sirloin)
- 1/3 cup almond meal
- 1 egg, beaten
- 1 tablespoon fresh mint, minced
- 1 teaspoon salt Pinch of cumin Soup
- 1 tablespoon olive oil or grapeseed oil
- 1/2 onion, finely chopped
- 2 garlic cloves, minced
- 2 boxes of chicken stock (or 8 cups of Homemade stock if you have it on hand)
- 2 gluten-free chicken bouillon cubes 1 can of tomatoes, chopped (reserve juices)
- 2 cups loosely chopped kale
- 4–6 baby carrots, sliced
- Salt and pepper for seasoning

Instructions:

1. Place all meatball ingredients in a large bowl and combine evenly with your hands. Form into meatballs, about 1 inch to 1 1/2-inches in diameter.
2. In a Dutch oven, sauté the onions in the oil until soft.
3. Add the garlic and continue sautéing an additional 3–5 minutes.
4. Add the chicken stock and bouillon cubes and bring to a boil, making sure the bouillon cubes dissolve thoroughly.
5. Place meatballs in the stock and bring to a boil again.
6. Skim the foam off the top of the soup occasionally.
7. Reduce the heat to medium-low, add in the tomatoes and reserved juices. Cover and simmer for 20 minutes.
8. Add in the kale and carrots, cover, and simmer for another 20–30 minutes, seasoning with salt and pepper if necessary.

Simple Beef & Portobello

Stew: Serves 4–6

Cooking time: 3 hours

Ingredient:

- 1 pound grass-fed beef stew meat, cut into chunks
- 1/2 teaspoon onion powder to season beef
- 1 yellow onion, loosely chopped
- 3 stalks celery, loosely chopped
- 1/2 cup loosely chopped carrots
- 8 ounces portobello mushroom caps, loosely chopped (about 3–4 portobello caps)
- 1 14-ounce can diced tomatoes
- 3 ounces tomato paste (1/2 can)
- 1/2 cup chicken stock
- 1 tablespoon red wine vinegar
- 1/2 teaspoon dried oregano
- 1/2 teaspoon dried thyme
- 1 teaspoon salt, plus more for seasoning
- 1/2 teaspoon ground pepper, plus more for seasoning

Instructions:

1. Season beef with onion powder. Brown on high heat in a sauté pan, searing each side of the beef chunks, about 3–4 minutes total.
2. Pour beef into slow cooker; add in all remaining ingredients.
3. Cook on low 8–10 hours or high 4–5 hours until stew is ready, season with additional salt and pepper to taste.

Mushroom Cream, Asparagus, and Onion Soup

Serves: 2 – 3

Ingredient:

- 1 pound asparagus 1 medium onion, chopped
- 1 pound cremini, baby Bella, or button mushrooms
- 1 1/2 cups chicken or vegetable broth
- 1 teaspoon salt
- 1/2 teaspoon freshly ground pepper
- 1/2 cup heavy cream

Instruction

1. Cut and discard the rough ends of the asparagus, usually the bottom 2–3 inches of the stalk.
2. Cut the remaining asparagus into 2-inch pieces.
3. In a steamer basket, steam the asparagus, onion, and mushrooms for 5–7 minutes, until tender.
4. Simultaneously, heat the chicken broth until boiling.
5. Remove from heat.
6. In a blender purée the vegetables, chicken broth, salt, and pepper for 3–4 minutes, until smooth.
7. Add in heavy cream and pulse to blend it in until smooth. Serve immediately

KETO DIET
What is Ketosis

Ketosis is a disorder in which the body creates molecules called ketones that are produced by the liver. It is designed to give cells and organs energy, and can substitute glucose as an alternative source of fuel.

The ketogenic diet, is also referred to as the keto diet, is not a fad diet focused on questionable nutritional science. It has been around since ancient times, using the diet as part of a holistic epilepsy treatment for ancient Greeks. In addition, over here in the States, in the 1920s, it was a known form of therapy for childhood epileptic seizures. Unfortunately, with its penchant for immediate effects, this natural method of treatment had to give way to the modern advances of pharmaceutical science.

Happily, the ketogenic diet has found its way back into the mainstream yet again and probably for very good reasons! You see, the basis of the diet is to essentially trigger your body's own fat-burning mechanisms in order to fuel what the body requires for energy throughout the day. Which means the fat you consume, as well as the fat stored in your body, have all become fuel reserves that your body can depend on! No wonder this diet really helps you lose weight, even for those stubborn and hard to lose fatty areas.

That may be one of the reasons you chose this book and looked into embarking on the ketogenic path to feel inner peace and be happy, or you may have learned stuff from your social circle about how the keto diet really normalizes blood sugar levels and optimizes your cholesterol readings, and you're fascinated.

How about stories of type 2 diabetes being reversed just through following this diet alone, as well as tales of certain cancers being

---

halted or the tumours shrinking due to the positive effects of the keto diet? We must also not forget the accompanying risk reduction of cardiovascular disease as a result of the diet!

BENEFIT OF KETOGENIC LIFESTYLE

The keto diet is an excellent motivational booster or reminder during instances when you feel down about your body system. While on the keto journey, when the going gets tough and throwing in the towel becomes a somewhat palatable option.

Don't give up! These are the benefit awaiting you at the end of the tunnel!

Natural hunger suppression

Like what has been elaborated previously, this feature of the keto diet comes in really handy when your goal is to achieve some weight loss. You can now do so without suffering from crazy hunger pangs.

Sustainable weight loss and maintenance

Weight loss makes us feel this inner peace. Another thing that has it going for the ketogenic diet is the fact that you practically do not have to watch out for any sudden weight rebounds or crazy weight gains if you keep on track with the diet. The mechanics of ketosis does not allow that to happen, and of course, we are talking about regular meals here, not seven or eight thousand calorie food plans which would definitely upset the weight loss process. You still can put on weight if you eat too much!

Clearer thoughts in the mind

Due to the neuroprotective benefits that ketones actually confer on the brain, one of the additional advantages of going keto would be experiencing a sharper and clearer mind. Thought processes are touched with more clarity, without the brain fog that is common for folks on processed carb-rich diets. Ketones are burning more efficiently as fuel also contributes to this enhanced mental clarity.

Experience better and more stable moods

When the body enters ketosis, the ketones generated for energy also help with the balance between two neurotransmitters that govern the brain: GABA, also known as gamma-aminobutyric acid, as well as glutamate. GABA serves to calm the brain down, while glutamate acts as a stimulant for the cerebral system. The trick to a healthy and happy brain is to keep these two substances incorrect balance, and ketones certainly help to achieve that end.

Improve energy levels and solve chronic fatigue

Instead of having roller coaster spikes in your energy levels, the ketone fueled body will allow you to experience increased energy levels that stay more or less constant as long as you have your meals when hunger hits. Chronic fatigue also becomes a non-issue due to the elevated levels of energy. Even if chronic fatigue is a symptom of other diseases, many find that though it does not go away entirely, the tiredness gets better on the keto diet. Get your

inflammation levels down

When you ensure that you have an adequate balance of omega-3 fats, these healthy polyunsaturated fats help to decrease the inflammatory response in the body system. This makes for good news to those who are suffering from chronic inflammatory diseases. Besides, the carb restriction would probably see your sugar intake coming way down, which will definitely help in reducing inflammation as well.

Improve your lipid panel readouts

Going keto should usually see your HDL cholesterol rise while the LDL cholesterol levels go the other way. There could be several cases where you can see changes in both HDL and LDL levels, leading to an overall rise in cholesterol levels. Some folks have expressed concern about this subject, and I would like to expand on this a little bit more. For those that go through a ketogenic diet, LDL and total cholesterol levels can be elevated, but this should not completely freak you out! Think about it this way: if your body has been metabolically compromised over the years of eating refined and sugary carbohydrates, the rise in cholesterol is actually a sign that the body is going through a period of healing to normalize metabolic function. LDL and total cholesterol levels appear to start tilting downward when the damage is fully repaired. The body of everyone is special and so is the time it takes for the repair to be carried out. Many can see results in months, while others may take a year or two to reach the optimum rates.

Less oxidative stress

The ketogenic diet is responsible for increasing the antioxidants present in the body, while also directly reducing the oxidation that is encountered by the body's mitochondria. With boosted antioxidant activity while on the keto diet, free radicals tend to have a harder time in inflicting oxidative damage on our bodies. Less oxidation usually means that our cells and organs function better and enjoy a longer shelf life. This also means that there could be a chance to prolong our longevity, since oxidation, being one of the prime reasons behind ageing, sees its activity being restrained to some extent while on the ketogenic diet. These are only some of the benefits which you will get to enjoy when you go keto. I would have loved to put in more information, especially where the ketogenic diet has had positive effects on diseases like cancer, polycystic ovary syndrome, non-alcoholic fatty liver disease, and neurodegenerative ailments like Parkinson's and Alzheimer's.

Here are recommended keto recipes diet for breakfast, lunch, and dinner.

BREAKFAST

SheetPanEggswithVeggiesandParmesan

Servings: 6

Prep Time: 5 minutes

Cook Time: 15 minutes

Ingredients:

- 12 large eggs, whisked
- Salt and pepper
- 1 small red pepper, diced
- 1 small yellow onion, chopped
- 1 cup diced mushrooms
- 1 cup diced zucchini
- 1 cup freshly grated parmesan cheese

Instructions:

1. Preheat the oven to 350°F and grease a rimmed baking sheet with cooking spray.
2. Whisk the eggs in a bowl with salt and pepper until frothy.
3. Stir in the peppers, onions, mushrooms, and zucchini until well combined.
4. Pour the mixture in the baking sheet and spread into an even layer.
5. Sprinkle with parmesan and bake for 12 to 15 minutes until the egg is set.
6. Let cool slightly, then cut into squares to serve.

Nutrition Info: 215 calories, 14g fat, 18.5g protein, 5g carbs, 1g fibre, 4g net carbs

Kale Avocado Smoothie

Servings: 1

Prep Time: 5 minutes

Cook Time: None

Ingredients:

- 1 cup fresh chopped kale
- ½ cup chopped avocado
- ¾ cup unsweetened almond milk
- ¼ cup full-fat yoghurt, plain
- 3 to 4 ice cubes
- 1 tablespoon fresh lemon juice
- Liquid stevia extract, to taste

Instructions:

1. Combine the kale, avocado, and almond milk in a blender.
2. Pulse the ingredients several times.
3. Add the remaining ingredients and blend until smooth.
4. Pour into a large glass and enjoy immediately.

Nutrition Info: 250 calories, 19g fat, 6g protein, 17.5g carbs, 6.5g fibre, 11g net carbs

Almond Butter Protein Smoothie

Servings: 1

Prep Time: 5 minutes

Cook Time: None

Ingredients:

- 1 cup unsweetened almond milk
- ½ cup full-fat yoghurt, plain
- ¼ cup vanilla egg white protein powder
- 1 tablespoon almond butter
- Pinch ground cinnamon
- Liquid stevia extract, to taste

Instructions:

1. Combine the almond milk and yoghurt in a blender.
2. Pulse the ingredients several times.
3. Add the remaining ingredients and blend until smooth.
4. Pour into a large glass and enjoy immediately.

Nutrition Info: 315 calories, 16.5g fat, 31.5g protein, 12g carbs, 2.5g fibre, 9.5g net carb

Beets and Blueberry Smoothie

Servings: 1

Prep Time: 5 minutes

Cook Time: None

Ingredients:

- 1 cup unsweetened coconut milk
- ¼ cup heavy cream
- ¼ cup frozen blueberries
- 1 small beet, peeled and chopped
- 1 teaspoon chia seeds
- Liquid stevia extract, to taste

Instructions:

1. Combine the blueberries, beets, and coconut milk in a blender.
2. Pulse the ingredients several times.
3. Add the remaining ingredients and blend until smooth. 4. Pour into a large glass and enjoy immediately.

Nutrition Info: 215 calories, 17g fat, 2.5g protein, 15g carbs, 5g fibre, 10g net carbs

Almond Butter Muffins

Servings: 12

Prep Time: 10 minutes

Cook Time: 25 minutes

Ingredients:

- 2 cups almond flour
- 1 cup powdered erythritol
- 2 teaspoons baking powder
- ¼ teaspoon salt
- ¾ cup almond butter, warmed
- ¾ cup unsweetened almond milk
- 4 large eggs

Instructions:

1. Preheat the oven to 350°F and line a muffin pan with paper liners.
2. Whisk the almond flour together with the erythritol, baking powder, and salt in a mixing bowl.
3. In a separate bowl, whisk together the almond milk, almond butter, and eggs.
4. Stir the wet ingredients into the dry until just combined.
5. Spoon the batter into the prepared pan and bake for 22 to 25 minutes until a knife inserted in the centre comes out clean.
6. Cool the muffins in the pan for 5 minutes then turn out onto a wire cooling rack.

Nutrition Info: 135 calories, 11g fat, 6g protein, 4g carbs, 2g fibre, 2g net. carbs

Classic Western Omelet

Servings: 1

Prep Time: 5 minutes

Cook Time: 10 minutes

Ingredients:

- 2 teaspoons coconut oil
- 3 large eggs, whisked
- 1 tablespoon heavy cream
- Salt and pepper
- ¼ cup diced green pepper
- ¼ cup diced yellow onion
- ¼ cup diced ham

Instructions:

1. Whisk together the eggs, heavy cream, salt and pepper in a small bowl.
2. Heat 1 teaspoon coconut oil in a small skillet over medium heat.
3. Add the peppers, onions, and ham then sauté for 3 to 4 minutes.
4. Spoon the mixture into a bowl and reheat the skillet with the rest of the oil.
5. Pour in the whisked eggs and cook until the bottom of the egg starts to set.
6. Tilt the pan to spread the egg and cook until almost set.
7. Spoon the veggie and ham mixture over half the omelette and fold it over.
8. Let the omelette cook until the eggs are set then serve hot.

Nutrition Info: 415 calories, 32.5g fat, 25g protein, 6.5g carbs, 1.5g fibre, 5g net carbs

Cinnamon Protein Pancakes

Servings: 4

Prep Time: 5 minutes

Cook Time: 15 minutes

Ingredients:

- 1 cup of canned coconut milk
- ¼ cup of coconut oil
- 8 large eggs
- 2 scoops (40g) egg white protein powder
- 1 teaspoon vanilla extract
- ½ teaspoon ground cinnamon
- Pinch ground nutmeg
- Liquid stevia extract, to taste

Instructions:

1. Combine the coconut milk, coconut oil, and eggs in a food processor.
2. Pulse the mixture several times then add the remaining ingredients.
3. Blend until smooth and well combined – adjust sweetness to taste.
4. Heat a nonstick skillet over medium heat.
5. Spoon in the batter, using about ¼ cup per pancake.
6. Cook until bubbles form on the surface of the batter then carefully flip.
7. Let the pancake cook until the underside is browned.
8. Transfer to a plate to keep warm and repeat with the remaining batter.

Nutrition Info: 440 calories, 38g fat, 22g protein, 5.5g carbs, 1.5g fibre, 4g net carbs

Sheet Pan Eggs with Ham and

PepperJack Servings: 6

Prep Time: 5 minutes

Cook Time: 15 minutes

Ingredients:

- 12 large eggs, whisked
- Salt and pepper
- 2 cups diced ham
- 1 cup shredded pepper jack cheese

Instructions:

1. Preheat the oven to 350°F and grease a rimmed baking sheet with cooking spray.
2. Whisk the eggs in a bowl with salt and pepper until frothy.
3. Stir in the ham and cheese until well combined.
4. Pour the mixture in the baking sheet and spread into an even layer.
5. Bake for 12 to 15 minutes until the egg is set.
6. Let cool slightly then cut into squares to serve.

Nutrition Info: 235 calories, 15g fat, 21g protein, 2.5g carbs, 0.5g fibre, 2g net carbs

Detoxifying Green Smoothie

Servings: 1

Prep Time: 5 minutes

Cook Time: None

Ingredients:

- 1 cup fresh chopped kale
- ½ cup fresh baby spinach
- ¼ cup sliced celery
- 1 cup water• 3 to 4 ice cubes
- 2 tablespoons fresh lemon juice
- 1 tablespoon fresh lime juice
- 1 tablespoon coconut oil
- Liquid stevia extract, to taste

Instructions:

1. Combine the kale, spinach, and celery in a blender.
2. Pulse the ingredients several times.
3. Add the remaining ingredients and blend until smooth.
4. Pour into a large glass and enjoy immediately.

Nutrition Info: 160 calories, 14g fat, 2.5g protein, 8g carbs, 2g fibre, 6g net carbs

Nutty Pumpkin Smoothie

Servings: 1

Prep Time: 5 minutes

Cook Time: None

Ingredients:

- 1 cup unsweetened cashew milk
- ½ cup pumpkin puree
- ¼ cup heavy cream
- 1 tablespoon raw almonds
- ¼ teaspoon pumpkin pie spice
- Liquid stevia extract, to taste

Instructions:

1. Combine all of the ingredients in a blender.
2. Pulse the ingredients several times, then blend until smooth.
   3. Pour into a large glass and enjoy immediately.

Nutrition Info: 205 calories, 16.5g fat, 3g protein, 13g carbs, 4.5g fibre, 8.5g net carbs

Tomato Mozzarella Egg Muffins

Servings: 12

Prep Time: 5 minutes

Cook Time: 25 minutes

Ingredients:

- 1 tablespoon butter
- 1 medium tomato, finely diced
- ½ cup diced yellow onion
- 12 large eggs, whisked
- ½ cup of canned coconut milk
- ¼ cup sliced green onion
- Salt and pepper
- 1 cup shredded mozzarella cheese

Instructions:

1. Preheat the oven to 350°F and grease a muffin pan with cooking spray.
2. Melt the butter in a medium skillet over medium heat.
3. Add the tomato and onions then cook for 3 to 4 minutes until softened.
4. Divide the mixture among the muffin cups.
5. Whisk together the eggs, coconut milk, green onions, salt, and pepper, then spoon into the muffin cups.
6. Sprinkle with cheese then bake for 20 to 25 minutes until the egg is set.

Nutrition Information: 135 calories, 10.5g fat, 9g protein, 2g carbs, 0.5g fibre, 1.5g net carbs

Crispy Chai Waffles

Servings: 4

Prep Time: 10 minutes

Cook Time: 20 minutes

Ingredients:

- 4 large eggs, separated into whites and yolks
- 3 tablespoons coconut flour
- 3 tablespoons powdered erythritol
- 1 ¼ teaspoon baking powder
- 1 teaspoon vanilla extract
- ½ teaspoon ground cinnamon
- ¼ teaspoon ground ginger
- Pinch ground cloves
- Pinch ground cardamom
- 3 tablespoons coconut oil, melted
- 3 tablespoons unsweetened almond milk

Instructions:

1. Separate the eggs into two different mixing bowls.
2. Whip the egg whites until stiff peaks form then set aside.
3. Whisk the egg yolks with the coconut flour, erythritol, baking powder, vanilla, cinnamon, cardamom, and cloves in the other bowl.
4. Add the melted coconut oil to the second bowl while whisking then whisk in the almond milk.
5. Gently fold in the egg whites until just combined.

6. Preheat the waffle iron and grease with cooking spray.
7. Spoon about ½ cup of batter into the iron.
8. Cook the waffle according to the manufacturer's instructions.
9. Remove the waffle to a plate and repeat with the remaining batter.

Nutrition Info: 215 calories, 17g fat, 8g protein, 8g carbs, 4g fibre, 4g net carbs

Broccoli Kale Egg Scramble

Servings: 1

Prep Time: 5 minutes

Cook Time: 10 minutes

Ingredients:

- 2 large eggs, whisked
- 1 tablespoon heavy cream
- Salt and pepper
- 1 teaspoon coconut oil
- 1 cup fresh chopped kale
- ¼ cup frozen broccoli florets, thawed
- 2 tablespoons grated parmesan cheese

Instructions:

1. Whisk the eggs together with the heavy cream, salt, and pepper in a bowl.
2. Heat 1 teaspoon coconut oil in a medium skillet over medium heat.
3. Stir in the kale and broccoli then cook until the kale is wilted, about 1 to 2 minutes.
4. Pour in the eggs and cook, occasionally stirring, until just set.
5. Stir in the parmesan cheese and serve hot.

Nutrition Info: 315 calories, 23g fat, 19.5g protein, 10g carbs, 1.5g fibre, 8.5g net carbs

LUNCH RECIPES

Cucumber Avocado Salad with Bacon

Servings: 2

Prep Time: 10 minutes

Cook Time: None

Ingredients:

- 2 cups fresh baby spinach, chopped
- ½ English cucumber, sliced thin
- 1 small avocado, pitted and chopped
- 1 ½ tablespoon olive oil
- 1 ½ tablespoon lemon juice
- Salt and pepper
- 2 slices cooked bacon, chopped

Instructions:

1. Combine the spinach, cucumber, and avocado in a salad bowl.
2. Toss with the olive oil, lemon juice, salt and pepper.
3. Top with chopped bacon to serve.

Nutrition Info: 365 calories, 24.5g fat, 7g protein, 13g carbs, 8g fibre, 5g net carbs

Bacon Cheeseburger Soup

Servings: 4

Prep Time: 10 minutes

Cook Time: 15 minutes

Ingredients:

- 4 slices uncooked bacon
- 8 ounces ground beef (80% lean)
- 1 medium yellow onion, chopped
- 1 clove garlic, minced
- 3 cups beef broth
- 2 tablespoons tomato paste
- 2 teaspoons Dijon mustard
- Salt and pepper
- 1 cup shredded lettuce
- ½ cup shredded cheddar cheese

Instructions:

1. Cook the bacon in a saucepan until crisp then drains on paper towels and chop.
2. Reheat the bacon fat in the saucepan and add the beef.
3. Cook until the beef is browned, then drain away half the fat.
4. Reheat the saucepan and add the onion and garlic – cook for 6 minutes.
5. Stir in the broth, tomato paste, and mustard then season with salt and pepper.
6. Add the beef and simmer on medium-low for 15 minutes, covered.
7. Spoon into bowls and top with shredded lettuce, cheddar cheese and bacon.

Nutrition Info: 315 calories, 20g fat, 27g protein, 6g carbs, 1g fibre, 5g net carbs

Ham and Provolone Sandwich

Servings: 1

Prep Time: 30 minutes

Cook Time: 5 minutes

Ingredients:

- 1 large egg, separated
- Pinch cream of tartar
- Pinch salt
- 1-ounce cream cheese softened
- ¼ cup shredded provolone cheese
- 3 ounces sliced ham

Instructions:

1. For the bread, preheat the oven to 300°F and line a baking sheet with parchment.
2. Beat the egg whites with the cream of tartar and salt until soft peaks form.
3. Whisk the cream cheese and egg yolk until smooth and pale yellow.
4. Fold in the egg whites a little at a time until smooth and well combined.
5. Spoon the batter onto the baking sheet into two even circles.
6. Bake for 25 minutes until firm and lightly browned.
7. Spread the butter on one side of each bread circle then place one in a preheated skillet over medium heat.
8. Sprinkle with cheese and add the sliced ham then top with the other bread circle, butter-side-up.
9. Cook the sandwich for a minute or two then carefully flip it over.
10. Let it cook until the cheese is melted then serve.

Nutrition Info: 425 calories, 31g fat, 31g protein, 5g carbs, 1g fibre, 4g net carbs

Baked Chicken Nuggets

Servings: 4

Prep Time: 10 minutes

Cook Time: 20 minutes

Ingredients:

- ¼ cup almond flour
- 1 teaspoon chilli powder
- ½ teaspoon paprika
- 2 pounds boneless chicken thighs, cut into 2-inch chunks
- Salt and pepper
- 2 large eggs, whisked well

Instructions:

1. Preheat the oven to 400°F and line a baking sheet with parchment.
2. Stir together the almond flour, chilli powder, and paprika in a shallow dish.
3. Season the chicken with salt and pepper, then dip in the beaten eggs.
4. Dredge the chicken pieces in the almond flour mixture, then arrange on the baking sheet.
5. Bake for 20 minutes until browned and crisp. Serve hot.

Nutrition Info: 400 calories, 26g fat, 43g protein, 2g carbs, 1g fibre, 1g net carbs

Taco Salad with Creamy Dressing

Servings: 2

Prep Time: 10 minutes

Cook Time: 10 minutes

Ingredients:

- 6 ounces ground beef (80% lean)
- Salt and pepper
- 1 tablespoon ground cumin
- 1 tablespoon chilli powder• 4 cups fresh chopped lettuce
- ½ cup diced tomatoes
- ¼ cup diced red onion
- ¼ cup shredded cheddar cheese
- 3 tablespoons mayonnaise
- 1 teaspoon apple cider vinegar
- Pinch paprika

Instructions:

1. Cook the ground beef in a skillet over medium-high heat until browned.
2. Drain half the fat, then season with salt and pepper and stir in the taco seasoning.
3. Simmer for 5 minutes, then remove from heat.
4. Divide the lettuce between two salad bowls, then top with ground beef.
5. Add the diced tomatoes, red onion, and cheddar cheese.
6. Whisk together the remaining ingredients, then drizzle over the salads to serve.

Nutrition Info: 470 calories, 36g fat, 28g protein, 7.5g carbs, 1.5g fibre, 6g net carbs

Egg Salad Over Lettuce

Servings: 2

Prep Time: 10 minutes

Cook Time: None

Ingredients:

- 3 large hardboiled eggs, cooled
- 1 small stalk celery, diced
- 3 tablespoons mayonnaise
- 1 tablespoon fresh chopped parsley
- 1 teaspoon fresh lemon juice
- Salt and pepper
- 4 cups fresh chopped lettuce

Instructions:

1. Peel and dice the eggs into a mixing bowl.
2. Stir in the celery, mayonnaise, parsley, lemon juice, salt and pepper.
3. Serve spooned over fresh chopped lettuce.

Nutrition Info: 260 calories, 23g fat, 10g protein, 4g carbs, 1g fibre, 3g net carbs

Egg Drop Soup

Servings: 4

Prep Time: 5 minutes

Cook Time: 10 minutes

Ingredients:

- 5 cups chicken broth
- 4 chicken bouillon cubes
- 1 ½ tablespoons chilli garlic paste
- 6 large eggs, whisked
- ½ green onion, sliced

Instructions:

1. Crush the bouillon cubes and stir into the broth in a saucepan.
2. Bring it to a boil, then stir in the chilli garlic paste.
3. Cook until steaming, then remove from heat.
4. While whisking, drizzle in the beaten eggs.
5. Let sit for 2 minutes then serve with sliced green onion.

Nutrition Info: 165 calories, 9.5g fat, 16g protein, 2.5g carbs, 0g fibre, 2.5g carbs

Bacon, Lettuce, Tomato, Avocado Sandwich

Servings: 1

Prep Time: 30 minutes

Cook Time: None

Ingredients:

- 1 large egg, separated
- Pinch cream of tartar
- Pinch salt
- 1-ounce cream cheese softened
- 2 slices uncooked bacon
- ¼ cup sliced avocado
- ¼ cup shredded lettuce
- 1 slice tomato

Instructions:

1.   For the bread, preheat the oven to 300°F and line a baking sheet with parchment.
2.   Beat the egg whites with the cream of tartar and salt until soft peaks form.
3.   Whisk the cream cheese and egg yolk until smooth and pale yellow.
4.   Fold in the egg whites a little at a time until smooth and well combined.
5.   Spoon the batter onto the baking sheet into two even circles.
6.   Bake for 25 minutes until firm and lightly browned.
7.   Cook the bacon in a skillet until crisp, then drain on a paper towel.
8.   Assemble the sandwich with the bacon, avocado, lettuce, and tomato.

Nutrition Info: 355 calories, 30g fat, 16.5g protein, 5.5g carbs, 2.5g fibre, 3g net carbs

Fried Salmon Cakes

Servings: 2

Prep Time: 15 minutes

Cook Time: 10 minutes

Ingredients:

- 1 tablespoon butter
- 1 cup riced cauliflower
- Salt and pepper
- 8 ounces boneless salmon fillet
- ¼ cup almond flour
- 2 tablespoons coconut flour
- 1 large egg
- 2 tablespoons minced red onion
- 1 tablespoon fresh chopped parsley
- 2 tablespoons coconut oil

Instructions:

1. Melt the butter in a skillet over medium heat, then cook the cauliflower for
2. 5 minutes until tender – season with salt and pepper.
3. Spoon the cauliflower into a bowl and reheat the skillet.
4. Add the salmon and season with salt and pepper.
5. Cook the salmon until just opaque, then remove and flake the fish into a bowl.
6. Stir in the cauliflower along with the almond flour, coconut flour, egg, red onion, and parsley.
7. Shape into 6 patties then fries in coconut oil until both sides are browned. **Nutrition Info:** 505 calories, 37.5g fat, 31g protein, 14.5g carbs, 8g fibre, 6.5g net carbs

DINNER RECIPES

Grilled Pesto Salmon with Asparagus

Servings: 4

Prep Time: 5 minutes

Cook Time: 15 minutes

Ingredients:

- 4 (6-ounce) boneless salmon fillets
- Salt and pepper
- 1 bunch asparagus, ends trimmed
- 2 tablespoons olive oil
- ¼ cup basil pesto

Instructions:

1. Preheat a grill to high heat and oil the grates.
2. Season the salmon with salt and pepper, then spray with cooking spray.
3. Grill the salmon for 4 to 5 minutes on each side until cooked through.
4. Toss the asparagus with oil and grill until tender, about 10 minutes.
5. Spoon the pesto over the salmon and serve with the asparagus.

Nutrition Info: 300 calories, 17.5g fat, 34.5g protein, 2.5g carbs, 1.5g fibre,

1g net carbs

Cheddar-Stuffed Burgers with Zucchini

Servings: 4

Prep Time: 10 minutes

Cook Time: 15 minutes

Ingredients:

- 1 pound ground beef (80% lean)
- 2 large eggs
- ¼ cup almond flour
- 1 cup shredded cheddar cheese
- Salt and pepper
- 2 tablespoons olive oil
- 1 large zucchini, halved and sliced

Instructions:

1. Combine the beef, egg, almond flour, cheese, salt, and pepper in a bowl.
2. Mix well, then shape into four even-sized patties.
3. Heat the oil in a large skillet over medium-high heat.
4. Add the burger patties and cook for 5 minutes until browned.
5. Flip the patties and add the zucchini to the skillet, tossing to coat with oil.
6. Season with salt and pepper and cook for 5 minutes, stirring the zucchini occasionally.
7. Serve the burgers with your favourite toppings and the zucchini on the side.

Nutrition Info: 470 calories, 29.5g fat, 47g protein, 4.5g carbs, 1.5g fibre, 3g net carbs

Chicken Cordon Bleu with Cauliflower

Servings: 4

Prep Time: 10 minutes

Cook Time: 45 minutes

Ingredients:

- 4 boneless chicken breast halves (about 12 ounces)
- 4 slices deli ham• 4 slices Swiss cheese
- 1 large egg, whisked well
- 2 ounces pork rinds
- ¼ cup almond flour
- ¼ cup grated parmesan cheese
- ½ teaspoon garlic powder
- Salt and pepper
- 2 cups cauliflower florets

Instructions:

1. Preheat the oven to 350°F and line it with a foil baking sheet.
2. Sandwich the chicken breast halves between pieces of parchment and pound flat.
3. Lay the pieces out and top with sliced ham and cheese.
4. Roll the chicken up around the fillings then dip in the beaten egg.
5. Combine the pork rinds, almond flour, parmesan, garlic powder, salt and pepper in a food processor and pulse into fine crumbs.
6. Roll the chicken rolls in the pork rind mixture then place on the baking sheet.
7. Toss the cauliflower with melted butter then add to the baking sheet.
8. Bake for 45 minutes until the chicken is cooked through.

Nutrition Info: 420 calories, 23.5g fat, 45g protein, 7g carbs, 2.5g fibre, 4.5g net carbs

Sesame-Crusted Tuna with Green Beans

Servings: 4

Prep Time: 15 minutes

Cook Time: 5 minutes

Ingredients:

- ¼ cup white sesame seeds
- ¼ cup black sesame seeds
- 4 (6-ounce) ahi tuna steaks
- Salt and pepper
- 1 tablespoon olive oil
- 1 tablespoon coconut oil
- 2 cups green beans

Instructions:

1. Combine the two types of sesame seeds in a shallow dish.
2. Season the tuna with salt and pepper.
3. Dredge the tuna in the sesame seed mixture.
4. Heat the olive oil in a skillet to high heat then add the tuna.
5. Cook for 1 to 2 minutes until seared then turn and sear on the other side.
6. Remove the tuna from the skillet and let the tuna rest while you reheat the skillet with the coconut oil.
7. Fry the green beans in the oil for 5 minutes then serve with sliced tuna.

Nutrition Info: 380 calories, 19g fat, 44.5g protein, 8g carbs, 3g fibre, 5g net carbs

Rosemary Roasted Pork with Cauliflower

Servings: 4

Prep Time: 10 minutes

Cook Time: 20 minutes

Ingredients:

- 1 ½ pound boneless pork tenderloin
- 1 tablespoon coconut oil
- 1 tablespoon fresh chopped rosemary
- Salt and pepper
- 1 tablespoon olive oil
- 2 cups cauliflower florets

Instructions:

1. Rub the pork with coconut oil, then season with rosemary, salt, and pepper.
2. Heat the olive oil in a large skillet over medium-high heat.
3. Add the pork and cook for 2 to 3 minutes on each side until browned.
4. Sprinkle the cauliflower in the skillet around the pork.
5. Reduce the heat to low, then cover the skillet and cook for 8 to 10 minutes until the pork is cooked through.
6. Slice the pork and serve with the cauliflower.

Nutrition Info: 300 calories, 15.5g fat, 37g protein, 3g carbs, 1.5g fibre, 1.5g net carbs

Chicken Tikka with Cauliflower Rice

Servings: 6

Prep Time: 10 minutes

Cook Time: 6 hours

Ingredients:

- 2 pounds boneless chicken thighs, chopped
- 1 cup of canned coconut milk
- 1 cup heavy cream
- 3 tablespoons tomato paste
- 2 tablespoons garam masala
- 1 tablespoon fresh grated ginger
- 1 tablespoon minced garlic
- 1 tablespoon smoked paprika
- 2 teaspoons onion powder
- 1 teaspoon guar gum
- 1 tablespoon butter
- 1 ½ cup riced cauliflower

Instructions:

1. Spread the chicken in a slow cooker, then stir in the remaining ingredients except for the cauliflower and butter.
2. Cover and cook on low heat for 6 hours until the chicken is done and the sauce thickened.
3. Melt the butter in a saucepan over medium-high heat.
4. Add the riced cauliflower and cook for 6 to 8 minutes until tender.
5. Serve the chicken tikka with the cauliflower rice.

Nutrition Info: 485 calories, 32g fat, 43g protein, 6.5g carbs, 1.5g fibre, 5g net carbs

Grilled Salmon and Zucchini with Mango Sauce

Servings: 4

Prep Time: 5 minutes

Cook Time: 10 minutes

Ingredients:

- 4 (6-ounce) boneless salmon fillets
- 1 tablespoon olive oil
- Salt and pepper
- 1 large zucchini, sliced in coins
- 2 tablespoons fresh lemon juice
- ½ cup chopped mango
- ¼ cup fresh chopped cilantro
- 1 teaspoon lemon zest
- ½ cup of canned coconut milk

Instructions:

1. Preheat a grill pan to high heat and spray liberally with cooking spray.
2. Brush the salmon with olive oil and season with salt and pepper.
3. Toss the zucchini with lemon juice and season with salt and pepper.
4. Place the salmon fillets and zucchini on the grill pan.
5. Cook for 5 minutes then turn everything and cook 5 minutes more.
6. Combine the remaining ingredients in a blender and blend into a sauce.
7. Serve the salmon fillets drizzled with the mango sauce and zucchini on the side.

Nutrition Info: 350 calories, 21.5g fat, 35g protein, 8g carbs, 2g fibre, 6g net carbs

Slow-Cooker Pot Roast with Green Beans

Servings: 8

Prep Time: 10 minutes

Cook Time: 8 hours

Ingredients:

- 2 medium stalks celery, sliced
- 1 medium yellow onion, chopped
- 1 (3-pound) boneless beef chuck roast
- Salt and pepper
- ¼ cup beef broth
- 2 tablespoons Worcestershire sauce
- 4 cups green beans, trimmed
- 2 tablespoons cold butter, chopped

Instructions:

1. Combine the celery and onion in a slow cooker.
2. Place the roast on top and season liberally with salt and pepper.
3. Whisk together the beef broth, and Worcestershire sauce then pour it in.
4. Cover and cook on low heat for 8 hours until the beef is very tender.
5. Remove the beef to a cutting board and cut into chunks.
6. Return the beef to the slow cooker and add the beans and chopped butter.
7. Cover and cook on high for 20 to 30 minutes until the beans are tender.

Nutrition Info: 375 calories, 13.5g fat, 53g protein, 6g carbs, 2g fibre, 4g net carbs

PLEASE DON'T BE SO HASTY

Besides, slow eating speed can make you happier in the long run, especially those who want to lose weight. Several studies show a direct connection between the pace of eating and the development of obesity.

If the meal is "hastily swallowed dow", there is a risk of eating more than necessary, i.e. too much, in the time allotted for eating. With a moderate eating speed and thorough chewing of the food, on the other hand, the feeling of satiety is already appropriate during eating and hunger.

Also, the eating process requires our undivided attention. Eating and reading or watching TV at the same time can have a negative impact on the taste and speed of eating.

With the following tips, meals are a pleasure:

- Relax: Prepare or select the dishes consciously, lay the table and come to rest are important rituals to get in the mood for the food.
- Take your time: This includes sufficient time for a quiet breakfast and lunch break.
- Eat slowly: The feeling of satiety only sets in after a few minutes. Those who take their time eating are more likely to feel full - and automatically eat less.
- Chew thoroughly: The food is only opened up by sufficient chewing so that the body can digest the ingested food more easily and utilize the nutrients better.
- Without distraction: Those who only focus on eating perceive important body signals much more clearly, such as the beginning feeling of satiety. So better leave the TV out.
- Enjoy: Eating with all your senses conveys well-being. If you like to enjoy together, you can plan a picnic with the

family or brunch with friends at the weekend for a change.

- Do it yourself: Cooking promotes not only the senses and enjoyment but also the appreciation of our food. Cooking with children is particularly important. In childhood, the course is set early for healthy eating behaviour.

CPSIA information can be obtained
at www.ICGtesting.com
Printed in the USA
LVHW081816010621
689062LV00015B/1800

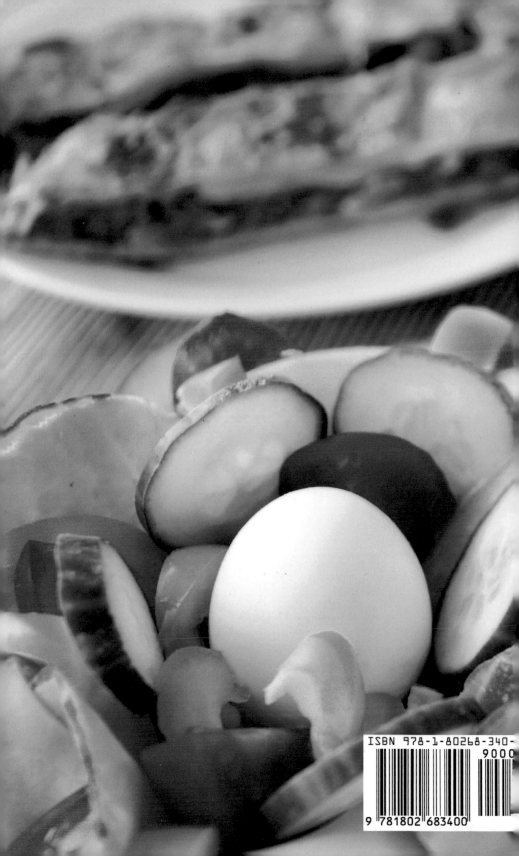

ISBN 978-1-80268-340-

9000

9 781802 683400

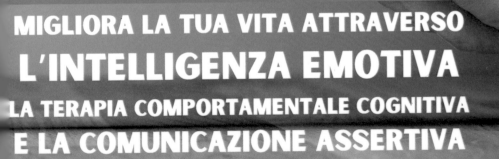

Mind Change Academy

CRESCITA PERSONALE

3 Libri in 1

**MIGLIORA LA TUA VITA ATTRAVERSO
L'INTELLIGENZA EMOTIVA
LA TERAPIA COMPORTAMENTALE COGNITIVA
E LA COMUNICAZIONE ASSERTIVA**